MY BARI TALE

The ultimate self-help guide to mentally prepare for bariatric surgery and to create new habits for success

CONTENT

-01-

NOT THE EASY WAY OUT

Helping you manage self-limiting beliefs and dealing with the bariatric surgery stigma.

-02-

MY PRE-OP JOURNEY

Documenting all of the things that matter during your pre-op stage. From pre-op appointments to your hospital bag checklist. It's all here.

-03-

MY FIRST YEAR POST-OP

Focus on your recovery. Learn how to deal with post-op challenges. And finally, create new habits that last way beyond your honeymoon stage.

-04-

MONTHLY HABIT TRACKERS

Now that you've learned how to create new habits - it's time to do the work. And keep track of them for the next 12 months of your journey.

-05-

QUARTERLY PROGRESS CHARTS

Measure your progress on and off the scale in month 3, month 6, month 9 and month 12 of your journey.

DISCLAIMER

**Share your bari-tale with us on our socials.
We're a community - you're not alone!**

www.youronederland.com
www.bari-tasty.com

 @your.onederland

 @bariatric.surgery.squad

@bariatric.surgery.squad

Disclaimer

This journal is made for educational, entertaining and inspirational purposes only and is not intended as personal or medical advice.

By reading this document, the reader acknowledges that the information provided in this book is not intended as nutritional, clinical, medical, legal or financial advice. Always consult a licensed specialist before attempting any techniques presented in this book.

All effort has been made to provide correct, accurate and up to date information. No warranties of any kind are declared or implied.

By reading this document, the reader agrees that under no circumstances the author is responsible for any direct or indirect losses, as a result of the use of information of this document, including but not limited to inaccuracies, omissions or errors of any kind.

A BARI-TALE

The pale green paint was slowly coming off the walls. And there was a clinical feel to this room. No wonder, because Mary was in the dietitian's office in a clinic nearby her house. Her mother insisted on taking her there. She just turned 6 years old.

Mary always felt like she was different. The "odd one". As the youngest sibling of three, Mary didn't have the genetics her older sisters had. You know, that perfect bone structure, an hourglass figure and the seemingly miraculous metabolism that made them able to eat anything they want, without gaining a single pound.

That wasn't her.

Mary was struggling with her weight for as long as she could remember. Or at least, it became even more of a struggle for her, because other people were so obsessed with it.

And just like every child's inner voice is a result of its caregivers outer voice - it didn't take long for Mary to perceive herself the way others did.

"Don't let Mary see that cake! She'll probably eat it all!"

"Is Mary supposed to eat that? It'll only make her fatter than she already is".

"Mary, Mary, has a big wobble-belly!"

The voices remained an echo in her ears for many years to follow. And in the back of her mind and the depths of her heart, she felt like a failure.

Fast forward 20 years later. Mary graduated from a decent college and got herself a decent job. She was engaged to the love of her life. She should be feeling happy right now. But in all honesty, she wasn't.

A lifelong battle with her weight has caused her self-esteem to plummet. And years of yo-yo dieting didn't do any good for her relationship with food either. She hated the way she looked. She hated every single picture with her in it. She didn't feel like she deserved to feel happiness.

But it wasn't until 1 year after her engagement, that Mary took the leap of faith and opened a new chapter in her life.

Her bariatric journey began.

CHANGING THE NARRATIVE OF YOUR OWN STORY

You're not Mary. Your story may not even remotely resemble hers. But one thing is for certain. Making the decision to have bariatric surgery is courageous, and here's why:

- Resizing your stomach literally forces you to eat differently
- Eating differently forces you to examine your relationship with food
- Examining your relationship with food opens new doors to change your habits for good

And now comes the hard part.

Bariatric surgery doesn't automatically changes your mindset. That's the work that YOU are putting in.

And this journal can be your guide in doing so.

By the end of this book you have learned to:

- Address your limiting beliefs that prevent you becoming your best self
- Bring to life the person you truly want to be
- Identify your new habits that support your long term goals after bariatric surgery
- Make an actionable plan to create consistency
- Trust yourself and your new tool to actually succeed this time around

This journal is packed with prompts to create awareness. Don't be surprised that it's going to be quite challenging to start writing down your true thoughts.. You have to dig deep - and you may feel a bit uncomfortable in doing so.

Don't give up.

Even if you use this journal only 1 minute a day, you ARE making progress.

Remember, small stomach - small steps.

We believe you can do this, okay?

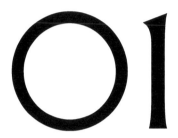

C H A P T E R

NOT THE EASY WAY OUT

Give yourself permission to embrace your journey. Because this is not the easy way out. And you're taking a courageous step towards reclaiming your own health, your life and your happiness.

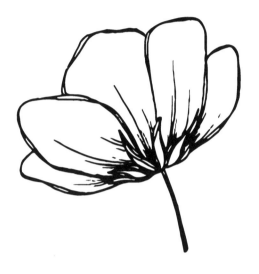

"

BARIATRIC SURGERY ISN'T THE EASY WAY OUT

IT'S JUST EASY TO SAY IT IS

-

YOUR ONEDERLAND

TO NEW BEGINNINGS

Real quick, this is how bariatric surgery works

Bariatric surgery is the generic name for all surgical procedures that change the digestive system in order to lose weight (and become healthier). The most common surgery procedures are the Vertical Sleeve Gastrectomy (VSG or Gastric Sleeve) and the Roux-en-Y Gastric Bypass (RNY or Gastric Bypass).

Some surgery procedures are solely restrictive, while others are malabsorptive too.

Bariatric surgery changes the way you digest food and it also changes your hunger hormones.

Also, by restricting the amount of food that you're able to eat in one sitting - a lower calorie intake is expected and weight loss follows.

This sounds quite logical right? And in theory it is. Bariatric surgery is an effective method. However, let's emphasize that every journey is different.

And not everyone will experience things like hunger, fullness and restriction the same way.

Also, bariatric surgery requires a specialized team to help you support your medical and nutritional goals too. Besides the physical part of surgery - it can be helpful to invest time in therapy too. Especially if you're overcoming food addiction or binge eating disorder.

You don't have to go through this alone - and never be ashamed to ask for help if you need it.

When all other attempts to lose weight in the past have failed

Bariatric surgery is the gold standard when it comes down to treating severe obesity. Up until this day, bariatric surgery is the most effective treatment for extreme overweight and its co-morbidities (other illnesses associated with the weight).

Now, does that mean that bariatric surgery is something to think lightly of? Absolutely not. Bariatric surgery is only the beginning of your journey. What comes next explains why bariatric is far from cheating.

Why bariatric surgery isn't a cop out

Having 80% of your stomach removed or bypassed - requires 100% commitment and hard work. Some days you'll feel on top the world. And sometimes, you don't even know where to start.

Because let's not forget about all the guidelines to commit to, like:

- Meeting your protein goals
- Staying hydrated
- Separating solids from liquids
- Eating slow, and of course;
- All the mindset work

Just because the weight comes off faster, doesn't mean that bariatric surgery is the easy way out.

And dealing with the bariatric stigma can be painful. It can be lonely when other people don't understand or support your decision to steer your life in a new direction.

But you know what?

Let them. You don't owe anyone an explanation for doing something that matters to you. Something that will help you change your relationship with yourself, with others and with food for once and for all.

Also, let's acknowledge that bariatric surgery is in fact, a last resort.

You probably tried every diet in the books. And you bought every "detox tea" out there - when you resorted to every FAD diet there ever was - only leaving you hopeless, incredibly hangry and probably a few pennies lighter too.

When you literally tried **everything** in your power to lose weight to become healthier - bariatric surgery can be your missing piece of the puzzle.

But remember, bariatric surgery only works, when you put in the work too.

So let's start with identifying your self-limiting beliefs. What thoughts set you back in becoming who you want to be? What's holding you back?

Are you ready? Let's begin!

I'm letting go of these thoughts to make sure that I will create the lifestyle that I deserve:

WHAT THE BARIATRIC STIGMA CAN LOOK LIKE

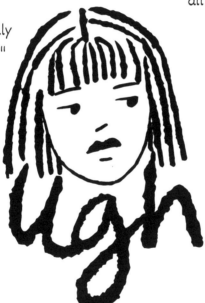

"But you're not even that big to have surgery"

"My neighbor gained all her weight back"

"Should you really be eating that?"

"Why don't you just go on a diet?"

"You're taking the easy way out"

"You're cheating"

Limiting beliefs that I catch myself on having are these:
Limiting beliefs are thoughts and feelings that sabotage your progress in any way or form. Write these down below.

....

....

....

....

....

....

....

....

....

....

....

....

....

The things that people said to me when I was judged for choosing bariatric surgery:

....

....

....

....

....

....

My ideal response to unsolicited comments is this:

....

....

....

....

....

....

....

....

This is on my mind right now:
This is free writing - jot down whatever comes to mind.

....

....

....

....

....

....

....

....

....

....

....

....

....

....

8 PILLARS TO REMEMBER

Success doesn't happen overnight. And while you're building a new lifestyle after bariatric surgery, it's important to keep 8 things in mind. Let's call these "things" the 8 mindset pillars that bridge the gap between your dreams and your success.

01

Small steps make all the difference

No habit is built overnight. Success is defined by taking small action every single day, consistently. The key to change isn't a glamorous event. But lies in the mundane day-to-day routines.

It's about drinking your water every day. It's about being mindful about eating slow every day. But the secret here isn't to be perfect. It's to start out as small as possible, so you can improve your habit along the way.

If you can't drink 8 glasses of water in a day right now. Then aim for drinking 1/2 glass more. And go from there. It's about the intention of showing up for yourself, however you can.

JOURNAL IT OUT

How can you make small changes today?

....

....

....

....

....

....

....

....

....

....

....

....

....

....

02

Take responsibility for your own actions

Although obesity is a complex disease where many variables that you simply can't control lay at the foundation of its complexity - it's still going to be important to take full responsibilty of the things you CAN control.

You can't control the genes you were born with. But you can control how much time you're going to spend on meal planning.

You can't control your body type, but you can control how much time you're going to spend on planning daily movement in your lifestyle.

Always own your actions. It will make you humble and stronger.

....

....

....

....

....

....

....

....

JOURNAL IT OUT

What things do you need to own that you may feel guilty/shameful about?

Be honest. There's no right or wrong. Just growth.

....

....

....

....

....

....

....

03

Know what you want. Set specific goals.

It's so much harder to be successful in your bariatric journey if you haven't defined what "success" means to you.

Is it to get rid of certain medications? Is it to look in the mirror and love the reflection that's looking back at you? Is it to wear a specific clothing item because you know you feel amazing wearing it?

Make your goal(s) specific, so that you know exactly why you're working so hard (you'll write down your "why" in the next chapter too).

Remember, the sky is the limit. No goals are out of reach. Believe it.

JOURNAL IT OUT

What goals do you want to accomplish? Write them down below.

....

....

....

....

....

....

....

....

....

....

....

....

....

....

....

O4

Stop comparing your journey with someone else

Comparing journeys can already start in the pre-op phase. "Why didn't I lose more weight during my pre-op diet?" "Why did it take so long for MY surgery to get approved, but hers was decided in a blink of an eye?"

And after surgery comparison can truly be the thief of your joy. It's best to already engrain this reminder in your mindset, right now. It's only human to compare, but don't let it become a pitfall that creates more doubts and insecurities.

We'll talk about that in the next pillar!

JOURNAL IT OUT

How are you making sure that you're going to focus on YOURSELF? How are you protecting your energy from the pitfall of comparison?

05

Visualize your goals. Every single day again.

Now that you've put your goals in writing, it's time to create a vision to bring your "new" you to life.

And now comes the hard part too. You have to believe that you can actually reach your goals. You have to put your doubts, fears and feelings of failure aside to start living like you've already accomplished what you're striving for. If you find this challenging, use the "fear shredder" in the next chapter to address your greatest fears.

Don't let any insecurities get in the way of becoming who you truly want to be. Because you deserve it.

JOURNAL IT OUT

Write your vision down in words. How do you feel? Whom are you with? What are you doing? How do you look? Visualize your best self and put it in writing.

MY BARIATRIC VISION BOARD

"This is how I envision myself and my life after bariatric surgery. This is who I want to be from now on. This is what inspires me. This is what motivates me. I'm using text, colors, images and whatever visual that I find helpful to make my vision board."

MY BARIATRIC VISION BOARD

O6

Accept the fact that you have to make sacrifices

Every form of success comes with a sacrifice. If you want to be a successful writer, you have to sacrifice your time.
If you want to invest in a new car, you have to sacrifice your money.

And if you want to be successful after bariatric surgery you'll have to sacrifice the things that prevent you from achieving your goals. Or to sacrifice the means to get you there.

Examples are: sacrificing certain trigger foods as a coping mechanism. Or sacrificing your time so that you can plan your meals ahead.

If you're not willing to give up some of your 'old' habits - success will be nearly impossible to maintain.

JOURNAL IT OUT

What are the things you need to sacrifice to achieve your goals after bariatric surgery? And through which means can you achieve your goals better?

....

....

....

....

....

....

....

....

....

....

....

....

....

....

....

O7

Face your fears. And do it anyway.

The only way to achieve long-term success after bariatric surgery is by overcoming your doubts and insecurities. That doesn't mean that you aren't allowed to feel them. Feelings are normal, they're okay and they're part of being human. But what can't get in the way of you achieving your goals - is the feeling of failure..

Fear is paralyzing and can make you apathetic - not having the energy to move forward. Fear is what holds you back in standing up for yourself and claiming YOUR wants and needs.

Use the fear shredder in the next section to shred your fears. And start with writing them down here as well.

JOURNAL IT OUT

Which fears get in the way of reaching your goals? Think about a time in your life that you were afraid, but made the leap of faith anyway. Hold on to that.

....

....

....

....

....

....

....

....

....

....

....

....

....

....

....

O8

Accept the fact that you made a commitment. A commitment for the rest of your life.

Bariatric surgery doesn't have a magical finish line. Your journey doesn't end when you hit a new milestone. Committing to bariatric surgery means making several promises to yourself to continue the process of growth and self-improvement. For the rest of your life.

After much practice, habits do become more automated (and thus easier to act on). But there always needs to be a form of mindfulness in your journey.

Because it's so easy to "fall off track" when you stop paying attention to the habits that lead to success, right?

JOURNAL IT OUT

What promises are you making to yourself in this journey? Which non-negotiables are the most important to you - the ones you intend to keep for the rest of your life?

....

....

....

....

....

....

....

....

....

....

....

....

....

....

MY NOTES

....

....

....

....

....

....

....

....

....

....

....

....

....

....

CHAPTER

02

MY PRE-OP JOURNEY

Mindset work starts in your pre-op stage. You can never 100% prepare yourself for the unknown - but what you can do is put your best foot forward to start your new life with the right tools. In this chapter, you'll find journaling prompts, pre-op trackers and so much more to make the most out of your pre-op journey.

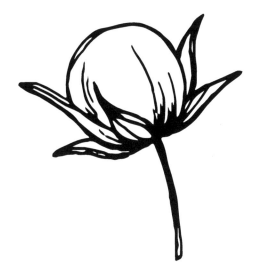

"

BARIATRIC SURGERY IS A MARATHON

NOT A SPRINT

-

YOUR ONEDERLAND

IT ALL BEGINS WITH THIS

A new lifestyle

Bariatric surgery isn't the start of a new diet – but the beginning of a whole new lifestyle. Sounds rather cliché, right? But that doesn't make it any less true.

"A new lifestyle". What does that even mean? And how do you start 'living that new life'?

Your bariatric journey kicks off long before your surgery day. And you already have a head start with your transformation, even before you lose your first pounds. Why? Because change starts within. It begins with your decision with bariatric surgery and the choice to reclaim your life.

Here are 5 things that go hand-in-hand with preparing for your surgery:

- Intentionally working towards changing your habits
- Working together with a bariatric team
- Learning about the bariatric surgery guidelines
- The pre-operative liquid diet
- Packing your hospital bag and learn what to expect during the first days post-op

Working together with a bariatric team

Bariatric surgery is more successful, safe and secure when you work closely with a bariatric team to support you. Not only your surgeon, but also a bariatric dietitian, a bariatric nurse, a trainer and a licensed therapist are often part of your multidisciplinary team to make your bariatric journey a success.

If you're paying your surgery out of pocket and following up with a bariatric team isn't mandatory - it's still strongly recommended to do so.

Because research shows that your post-op success is partly determined by the commitment to your follow-up appointments. And it not just boils down to success in terms of that number on the scale.

Yes, bariatric surgery is referred to as "minimum invasive surgery". But the physical and mental impact of having weight loss surgery should be taken seriously. With proper tools and the right support, you're putting both your physical and mental health in first place.

MY BARIATRIC BIO

Name: ....

Date of birth: ....

Height: ....

Highest weight: ....

Lowest weight: ....

My passion: ....

This is me

Type of surgery: ....

Surgery date: ....

My clinic / hospital: ....

My surgeon's name: ....

Emergency contact: ....

MY WHY

When things get tough, remember your why

Bariatric surgery isn't an impulsive decision without any decent thought to it. It takes months or even years to commit yourself to such a life-changing event. And you probably considered every pro and con, before taking that leap of faith too.

Now back to your "WHY".

Your "why" is going to be your main motivation when you feel like giving up. The reasons you want to change - are also the parts of your identity that you value the most.

For example, if one of the reasons is "to be able to freely participate in all social activities" - it's highly likely you consider yourself a social person. And that you value social events.

And if one of your "why's" is to "get rid of my medication" - then you value your health. And you want to become a "healthy person". Keep these thoughts in mind when you're going to envision your best self later on in this journal.

But first, let's start with writing down your "why" (and yes - you can write down ALL the reasons).

This is my why. This is my motivation. This is why I choose bariatric surgery:

....

....

....

....

....

MY WHY

....

....

....

....

....

....

....

....

....

....

....

....

....

PRE-OP THOUGHTS BEFORE BARIATRIC SURGERY BE LIKE

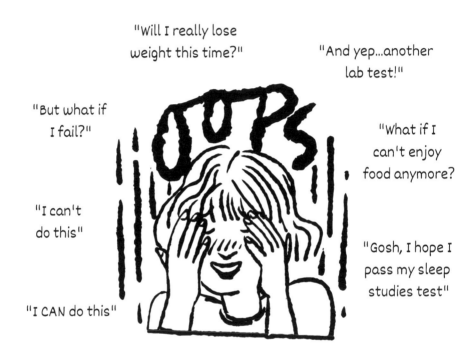

How to manage the fear of failure

It's normal to be scared of the unknown. It's normal to feel uncertain whether you're really going to be successful this time. When all attempts to lose weight didn't work in the past - it's completely normal to feel like this may not work as well.

But remember that things can be different now. Now, you have a tool at your disposal to help you change your lifestyle for good. A tool that you can use in your advantage with the right support, continuous effort and of course, self-compassion.

You can't control everything that happens in life. But what you can control is how you're going to put your best foot forward to make this journey a successful one.

BARIATRIC SURGERY ISN'T ANOTHER FAD DIET

IT'S A WHOLE NEW LIFESTYLE

These are my greatest fears before bariatric surgery:
Be honest about what worries you the most.

....

....

....

....

....

....

....

....

....

....

....

....

....

....

FEAR SHREDDER

**Use the dotted lines to describe each fear in one word.
Address them. Shred them.**

....

....

lessons

growth

opportunities

PREPARING FOR SURGERY

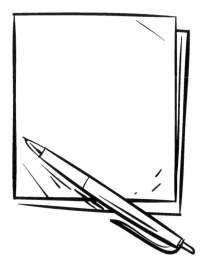

Below, you can find the pre-op section highlights.

PRE-OP APPOINTMENTS

Use the template in the next section to keep a close eye on all of your pre-op appointments leading up to your surgery day.

PRE-OP DIET

Use the pre-op diet tracker to prepare yourself for the pre-op diet. If you weren't prescribed a pre-op diet, use this tracker to begin with mindful eating.

HOSPITAL BAG ITEMS

Use the sample checklist as inspiration to pack your bag when leaving to have surgery.

MY HOSPITAL BAG

Fill in which must-haves you're going to bring with you to the hospital/clinic on your surgery day.

MY PRE-OP APPOINTMENTS

DATE | This is my appointment: | What I need to prepare:

DATE | This is my appointment: | What I need to prepare:

DATE | This is my appointment: | What I need to prepare:

DATE | This is my appointment: | What I need to prepare:

DATE | This is my appointment: | What I need to prepare:

DATE | This is my appointment: | What I need to prepare:

MY PRE-OP APPOINTMENTS

DATE | This is my appointment: | What I need to prepare:

DATE | This is my appointment: | What I need to prepare:

DATE | This is my appointment: | What I need to prepare:

DATE | This is my appointment: | What I need to prepare:

DATE | This is my appointment: | What I need to prepare:

DATE | This is my appointment: | What I need to prepare:

MY PRE-OP DIET

Start date: ....

End date: ....

Duration: ....

Calories: ....

Fat: ....

Carbs: ....

Protein: ....

Pre-op diet meal ideas:

Pre-op diet grocery list:

HOSPITAL BAG ITEMS

What are some of the most important essentials for your surgery day?
Below, you can find a sample checklist. And on the next page you can create your own list.

- ✔ comfortable underwear
- ✔ comfortable pj's
- ✔ phone extension cord
- ✔ phone charger
- ✔ lip balm
- ✔ medication
- ✔ warm socks
- ✔ comfortable slippers
- ✔ headphones
- ✔ wet wipes
- ✔ personal documents
- ✔ favorite playlist
- ✔ favorite movies/series
- ✔ thermos flask
- ✔ water bottles

- ✔ questions for your team
- ✔ flip-flops
- ✔ toiletries
- ✔ money & small change
- ✔ vaseline
- ✔ favorite pillow
- ✔ journal
- ✔ a pen
- ✔ mouth wash
- ✔ room spray
- ✔ incontinence pads
- ✔ plastic bags
- ✔ heating pad
- ✔ favorite books/magazine
- ✔ a scrunchy or bobby pins

MY HOSPITAL BAG

What I'm going to pack in my hospital bag:
No worries, you don't have to fill out the entire list. Just write down what you think is necessary to bring along with you. You'll probably overpack anyways!

✓ ....
✓ ....
✓ ....
✓ ....
✓ ....
✓ ....
✓ ....
✓ ....
✓ ....
✓ ....
✓ ....
✓ ....
✓ ....
✓ ....
✓ ....

✓ ....
✓ ....
✓ ....
✓ ....
✓ ....
✓ ....
✓ ....
✓ ....
✓ ....
✓ ....
✓ ....
✓ ....
✓ ....
✓ ....
✓ ....

A LETTER TO MYSELF

Dear me, this is what I want to tell you before starting this new journey:
Write down what you want to say to yourself before beginning this new chapter in your life. This is free writing, jot down whatever is important to you.

I SIMPLY CAN'T FAIL

BECAUSE I'M NEVER GIVING
UP ON MYSELF

MY FOOD FUNERAL

A food funeral is a ritual to say goodbye to old ways of eating and welcome the new. It's about letting go of consuming (large amounts of) trigger foods. This page isn't to favour the 'all-or-nothing mindset'. But rather to start your new chapter fresh. Use the dotted lines to write down your trigger foods.

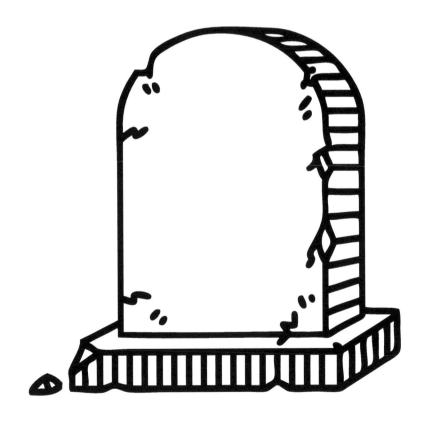

PRE-OP STAT CARD

Surgery date: ....

Highest weight: ....

Weight after pre-op diet: ....

Pre-op measurements:

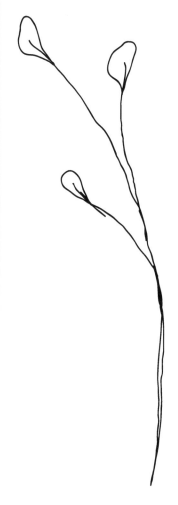

MY PRE-OP NOTES

THIS IS THE PRE-OP ME

HOW I FELT IN THIS PICTURE

....

....

....

CHAPTER

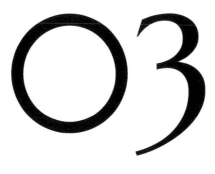

MY FIRST YEAR POST-OP

Healing after bariatric surgery is so much more than the mending of your incisions. It's about creating a balanced relationship with food, yourself and setting boundaries in your new lifestyle. A time for change.

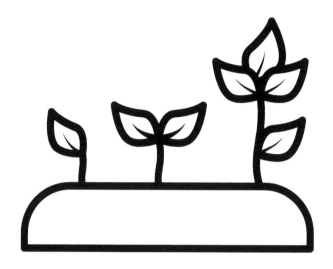

"

REMOVING OR BYPASSING 80% OF YOUR STOMACH - REQUIRES 100% OF YOUR COMMITMENT

-

YOUR ONEDERLAND

THE ROAD TO RECOVERY

After waking up from bariatric surgery

Bariatric surgery is life-changing, but that doesn't mean that it's going to be all sunshine and rainbows.

When you're in pain - and your life suddenly changes, there may be feelings of doubt and insecurity creeping in.

"What have I done?"

"Did I make the right decision?"

"Did I really just had 80% of my stomach surgically altered?"

Rest assured, "buyer's remorse" is fairly common in the first few weeks post-op.

Everything hurts. Everything is new. You're constantly worried whether that next sip will stay down this time. While also pondering on how you're going to meet your protein and hydration goals for the day.

It's a lot to deal with. And there's no bariatric fairy making that hardship during the first few days go away.

But at the same time, you're excited that your journey now really has begun (eek!).

This isn't going to be a walk in the park. It's going to be a whole lot of work. And we're going to help you follow through so that you can enjoy each and every milestone.

The key points in this chapter

In this chapter you'll learn how to start building your lifestyle after bariatric surgery. A lifestyle that's based on habits that support your post-op goals. A lifestyle that matches the person you envision yourself to be. You're going to build a new YOU with holding gratitude for the choices you made in the past.

Building habits is a crucial step to the road to recovery. Because bariatric surgery only works when you do. Bariatric surgery is only effective if YOU make the necessary lifestyle changes.

In this chapter you'll find a bariatric mood board and journaling prompts. And there's different bariatric trackers to help you meet your post-op goals more easily while focusing on the actual **process** (changing habits) to make the **progress** (the results).

POST-OP CHALLENGES ABC'S

But first, let's start with some of the most common post-op challenges. Bariatric surgery comes with many ups. But we can't forget about the daily struggles too. By acknowledging your challenges throughout your journey - you can find peace in learning new ways how to cope. Use the right column to write down how you navigate that specific challenge. If it doesn't affect you - simply tick off the box!

ALL-OR-NOTHING MINDSET

Ditching the all-or-nothing mindset can feel like an impossible task after - probably - years of dieting. But it's necessary to create more balance after bariatric surgery. Not all foods will fit, all the time. But eventually it's about creating a lifestyle where most of them will.
Tips: continue to work on your relationship with food after your surgery.

HOW I MANAGE

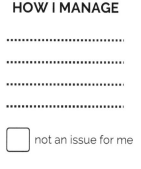

....

....

....

....

☐ not an issue for me

ODY DISTORTION

If you can't seem to grasp the physical transformation after you lost a significant amount of weight - you may find yourself experiencing body distortion. You still see the "old" you in the mirror.
Tips: look at your before and after pictures to see the physical changes. Consider therapy if you experience (signs) of body distortion or even body dysmorphia.

HOW I MANAGE

....

....

....

....

☐ not an issue for me

OMPARISON

It can be frustrating to see others lose weight quicker than you. Or to see other people who had the same surgery floating through their post-op life "effortlessly" (or so it seems). There's no such thing. Everybody has their own path to follow - and their own hurdles to tackle.
Tips: take a social media break - and focus on your own habits. Use your bariatric journal to create focus and more confidence.

HOW I MANAGE

....

....

....

....

☐ not an issue for me

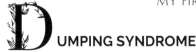

DUMPING SYNDROME

When (high-carb) food enter the small intestine too quickly - you may experience digestive issues like nausea, vomiting or diarrhoea. But dumping syndrome may also result in lower blood sugar levels leading to heart palpitations, dizziness and extreme fatigue.
Tips: eat slow, separate solids and liquids and be mindful about (too many) refined sugars.

HOW I MANAGE

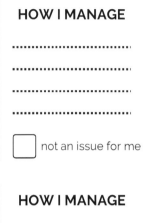

....

....

....

....

☐ not an issue for me

EATING OUT

Eating out can feel terrifying. Because what happens if you don't feel well? Or what if you can't focus on portion control? Or what would other people think when they see that you can't eat "that" much?
Tips: look up the menu before you go and decide at home, share your plate with a loved one, eat your protein first, order appetizers, order dressings on the side or request a 1/2 size portion.

HOW I MANAGE

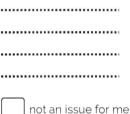

....

....

....

....

☐ not an issue for me

FULLNESS CUES

You may not recognize your fullness cues right away. Knowing when to stop eating is crucial to prevent overeating. Also, thinking that "one extra bite won't hurt" is going to backfire. It will.
Tips: fullness cues to look out for are sighing, burping, coughing, sneezing, hiccuping and the physical sensation of feeling full.

HOW I MANAGE

....

....

....

....

☐ not an issue for me

GRAZING

Nibbling on small amounts of (slider) foods* that don't keep you full for long, can lead to overeating and eventually - weight regain.
Tips: once you're on solids, try not to eat longer than 30 minutes (20 minutes would be ideal - because that's how long your brain needs to signal your pouch that you're full).

HOW I MANAGE

....

....

....

....

☐ not an issue for me

*Slider foods are foods that are high in simple carbs and low in protein or fiber. Learn more about slider foods in our free bariatric guide that can be downloaded here: www.youronederland.com/free-bariatric-guide

HAIR LOSS

Hair loss is common after bariatric surgery due to a swift change in hormones and the stress of surgery itself. Hair loss usually starts around 3 months post-op and is, for most, temporary.

Tips: eat your protein, take your daily vitamins and ask your surgeon if you need any additional supplements.

HOW I MANAGE

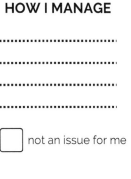

....

....

....

....

☐ not an issue for me

IRON DEFICIENCY

Foods that are rich in heme-iron*, aren't always tolerated well after bariatric surgery (for example, red meat).

Tips: do your lab work on time, take your vitamins, eat a high vitamin C food source with your iron based food sources (for example, spinach with steak). Legumes, like lentils, are high in (non-heme) iron too.

HOW I MANAGE

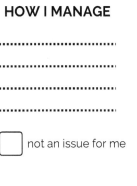

....

....

....

....

☐ not an issue for me

JOURNALING

Journaling - "I don't have time"
Watching series - "Finished 3 episodes in one go"
You get the gist right?

Tips: use your journal around the same time every day to turn it into a habit. Start small, even if you just write down a few words - it's a great start to keep the ball rolling.

HOW I MANAGE

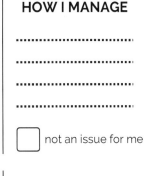

....

....

....

....

☐ not an issue for me

KINDNESS (TOWARDS YOURSELF)

Don't beat yourself up when you don't meet your goals. Give yourself grace even though the scale stops moving. Continue to show kindness towards yourself for making this commitment.

Tips: use positive affirmations, focus on your non-scale victories and use your journal to create self-awareness. Do more of what you love.

HOW I MANAGE

....

....

....

....

☐ not an issue for me

*Heme-iron is found in animal products like red meat. Non-heme iron is found in plant based food sources, such as spinach. Heme-iron is better absorbed than non-heme iron.

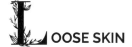

LOOSE SKIN

Loose skin isn't preventable most of the time because of rapid weight loss.
Tips: make exercise part of your lifestyle. It won't prevent loose skin altogether, but it's helpful for toning your body.

HOW I MANAGE

....
....
....
....

☐ not an issue for me

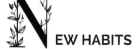

MEAL PLANNING

Planning your meals ahead will keep you focused on your post-op goals. It's a great habit to add to your post-op checklist.
Tips: start small - plan 1 meal ahead and see how that goes. Meal planning can be as simple as boiling 4 eggs in advance. Or prepping a container with your favorite high-protein snacks to-go.

HOW I MANAGE

....
....
....
....

☐ not an issue for me

NEW HABITS

This is probably the hardest part after bariatric surgery: creating new habits that last a lifetime. Habits will be your foundation for long-term success. Stay consistent.
Tips: start small - don't try to change everything at once (remember, the all-or-nothing mindset we want to get rid of?). Use your habit tracker to create consistency.

HOW I MANAGE

....
....
....
....

☐ not an issue for me

OBSESSING OVER THE SCALE

It can be SO easy to obsess over the number on the scale. Your weight is not your worth. And the scale doesn't measure your non-scale victories!
Tips: don't weigh yourself more than once a week. Or put the scale aside altogether and focus on creating your new habits we discussed in the previous section.

HOW I MANAGE

....
....
....
....

☐ not an issue for me

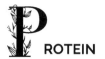PROTEIN

Protein is the key macronutrient after bariatric surgery. It helps with recovery and it prevents loss of muscle mass (together with exercise). Protein also curbs appetite.
Tips: eat your protein first with every meal, choose high-protein foods and spread your meals throughout the day to have more opportunities to get your protein in.

HOW I MANAGE

....
....
....
....

☐ not an issue for me

QUESTIONS

You may find yourself having a lot of questions after bariatric surgery. You're not alone - this is normal.
Tips: consult your bariatric team for personal advice. Seek reliable resources and join support groups to find comfort and a sense of togetherness.

HOW I MANAGE

....
....
....
....

☐ not an issue for me

REGAIN

One of the greatest fears after bariatric surgery: weight regain. A bit of regain is very normal - your lowest weight isn't always sustainable.
Tips: be mindful of grazing (the number 1 reason for weight regain) - and continue to work on your new habits. There's no finish line. You have to continue to show up for yourself (yes also, when you're getting closer to your goal weight).

HOW I MANAGE

....
....
....
....

☐ not an issue for me

STOMACH STRETCHING

Is it possible to stretch your new stomach? Theoretically, yes. It's normal that your stomach expands over time and that you're able to hold more food. Only a specialist can determine whether you've stretched your pouch beyond the norm.
Tips: separate solids and liquids, tune into your fullness cues and focus on protein and fiber as this maximizes your restriction.

HOW I MANAGE

....
....
....
....

☐ not an issue for me

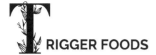

RIGGER FOODS

Bariatric surgery doesn't automatically fixes mind hunger or emotional eating. Some (trigger) foods won't fit in your lifestyle like the way they may have did before.
Tips: know what your trigger foods are and create awareness around your triggers (that may cause emotional eating). Consider therapy or more help if you continue to struggle in this area.

HOW I MANAGE

....
....
....
....

☐ not an issue for me

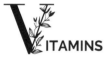

NDEREATING

If your restriction feels to high - you may find it challenging to meet your nutrient requirements. This could lead to undereating, grazing on slider foods and malnourishment.
Tips: consult your dietitian to create nourishing meals that fit your new lifestyle.

HOW I MANAGE

....
....
....
....

☐ not an issue for me

ITAMINS

One of the most important guidelines after bariatric surgery is taking your daily vitamins for the rest of your life. Which vitamins you need, depends on your type of surgery and your personal needs.
Tips: consult your surgeon about which vitamins are right for you.

HOW I MANAGE

....
....
....
....

☐ not an issue for me

EIGHT STALLS

When the scale stops moving - it can feel earth shattering. Rest assured. Stalls are normal. Sometimes the reason for a stall is within your control- and other times there's nothing you can do other than trust the process.
Tips: meet your protein goals, stay hydrated, focus on daily movement that you enjoy - take your vitamins. And work on your new mindset to manage disappointments.

HOW I MANAGE

....
....
....
....

☐ not an issue for me

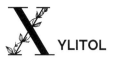
XYLITOL

Xylitol is a sugar alcohol that can be found in foods such as fruit. It's often used a sugar substitute. However, bariatric surgery can make you more sensitive to sugar alcohols in general. Good to know right?
 Tips: avoid foods that cause digestive issues. And re-introduce them to your diet with the help of your dietitian.

HOW I MANAGE

·····························
·····························
·····························
·····························

☐ not an issue for me

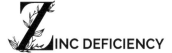
YOUR SUPPORT SYSTEM

Bariatric surgery is a personal journey. But having the right support is priceless. You're most likely to succeed if you have the right support post-op.
Tips: join support groups, find a supportive community, seek support from loved ones.

HOW I MANAGE

·····························
·····························
·····························
·····························

☐ not an issue for me

ZINC DEFICIENCY

An often overlooked deficiency after bariatric surgery: zinc. Signs of a zinc deficiency are hair loss, diarrhea, irritability and loss of appetite.
Tips: add foods high in zinc to your post-op diet. And discuss this with your dietitian. Examples are: meat, seafood (especially oysters) and poultry.

HOW I MANAGE

·····························
·····························
·····························
·····························

☐ not an issue for me

MY NOTES

···
···
···

THESE ARE MY "FIRSTS"

When you start over, and have given another chance in life - you will experience things for the first time. Write them down so you'll never forget.

My first sips of liquid: ....

My first puréed meal: ....

My first soft food: ....

My first solid meal: ....

My first poop: ....

My first hair loss: ....

My first dumping: ....

My first victory: ....

My first time crying: ....

My first weigh-in: ....

My first happy moment: ....

My first anxious moment: ....

My first intimate moment: ....

Here you'll have space to create your own "first times" after bariatric surgery. What made an impact on you? What took you by surprise?

My first ....

My first ....

My first ....

My first ....

My first ....

This is **my experience** from the moment I opened my eyes from surgery until I left the hospital/clinic):

....

....

....

....

....

....

....

....

....

....

....

....

....

....

This is **how I felt** from the moment I opened my eyes from surgery until I left the hospital/clinic (continued):

DON'T BE AFRAID TO FAIL

YOU NOW HAVE A TOOL TO HELP YOU CHANGE YOUR HABITS FOR GOOD

BUILDING NEW HABITS

The road to recovery goes way beyond the mending of your incisions.

Bariatric surgery doesn't fix your relationship with food. Bariatric surgery doesn't fix any ineffective habits that stray away you away from your **true** goals. Bariatric surgery creates restriction and therefore forces you to eat differently.

It forces you to examine your relationship with food on a microscopical level.

But the real road to recovery starts when you start changing your mindset. When you start changing the habits you have shaped over the past decades.

In this section you'll focus on the habits that will break or make you live the true life you want to live. You'll learn how to create awareness about the things you do that are going to help you to be the person you want to be. And you'll also become mindful about the ones that don't (without beating yourself up about it).

You don't have to be perfect

Creating new habits is gradual progress that requires consistency, discipline and a whole lot of self-compassion.

Beating yourself up for not being where you are (yet), isn't going to be helpful.

With that thought in mind, we strongly encourage to practice self-compassion and gratitude on every step of the way.

You don't have to strive for perfection. The key to consistency is focusing on small changes every day. It's all about taking modest steps and repeat them as often as you can, until they become automated. Until these habits become part of your new beliefs. In other words, learn to feel fulfilled with small progress.

Remember, by imagining your best self, you're using a compelling strategy to create routines that last way beyond the honeymoon stage.

If you have a clear vision in mind of who you strive to be and the kind of lifestyle you feel fits you most - the next step is to identify the habits that support this vision. And to let go of the ones that don't (this is what people often call 'bad habits').

In this section we'll focus on laying the foundation on how to create your own set of habits so that you can stick to your goals and jump for joy every time you reach a new milestone.

*The 'honeymoon stage' is referred to as the first 12-18 months post-op where most excess weight is lost.

This is the person I want to be after bariatric surgery:
Examples are:
"I want to be someone who puts myself first"
"I want to be someone who cares about my health"
"I want to be someone who handles food triggers with strength and confidence"
You can combine existing traits and habits with the ones you want to build in your post-op life. Use as many varieties as you want.

I want to be someone who: ....

....

I want to be someone who: ....

....

I want to be someone who: ....

....

I want to be someone who: ....

....

I want to be someone who: ....

....

I want to be someone who: ....

....

I want to be someone who: ....

....

I want to be someone who: ....

....

I want to be someone who: ....

....

I want to be someone who: ....

....

I want to be someone who: ....

....

Now it's time to create goals to match "your best self". For example, if you want to be someone who puts her/himself/theirselves first, you may want to think of a goal that's related to "setting boundaries". When you're goal is to be "healthy", you'll need to define what "healthy" means to you. You get the gist, right?
These are the habits I need to build to become the person that I want to be:

This habit supports my best self:

....

....

....

....

....

This habit supports my best self:

....

....

....

....

....

This habit supports my best self:

....

....

....

....

....

This habit supports my best self:

....

....

....

....

....

This habit supports my best self:

....

....

....

....

....

This habit supports my best self:

....

....

....

....

....

This habit supports my best self:

....

....

....

....

....

This habit supports my best self:

....

....

....

....

....

This habit supports my best self:

....

....

....

....

....

This habit supports my best self:

....

....

....

....

....

This habit supports my best self:

....

....

....

....

....

This habit supports my best self:

....

....

....

....

....

OLD HABITS BE GONE

**Fill the balloons with old habits you want to let go of.
Release the old and bring in the new!**

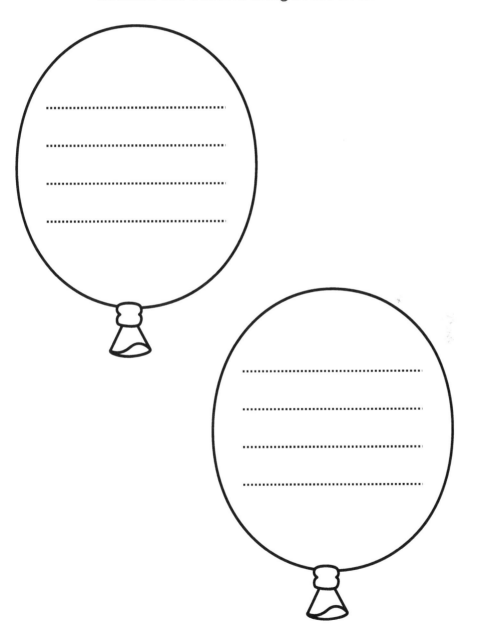

OLD HABITS BE GONE

**Fill the balloons with old habits you want to let go of.
Release the old and bring in the new!**

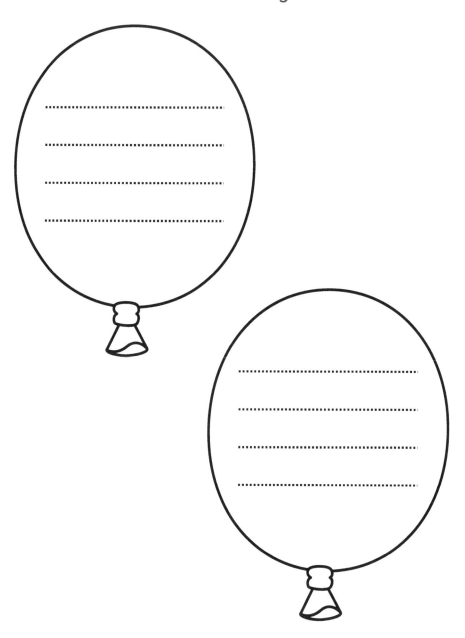

MY OWN PLAN

Now it's time to make a plan of action.
Create 1 plan per habit. Use this page as an example
for the habits you created earlier.

NEW HABIT

Planning meals ahead

HOW I'M GOING TO DO IT

Do groceries on Mondays. Write down my own meal plan for the next

day between 8-9 pm, every day. I will hold myself accountable by

using a planner. I will look up new recipes to feel inspired.

HOW I'M GOING TO MAKE THIS EASIER FOR MYSELF

I will start with eating the same breakfast every day - so I don't

have to think about too many different varieties just yet.

I will start with planning one meal per day. If that goes well, I'll plan

2 meals next. I won't try to be perfect. Just better than yesterday.

I will buy nice meal prep containers (just for myself) to make this

more enjoyable.

MY OWN PLAN

How are you going to change your habits in your day-to-day routine? How are you going to make it easier for yourself in doing so?

NEW HABIT

HOW I'M GOING TO DO IT

HOW I'M GOING TO MAKE THIS EASIER FOR MYSELF

MY OWN PLAN

How are you going to change your habits in your day-to-day routine? How are you going to make it easier for yourself in doing so?

NEW HABIT

HOW I'M GOING TO DO IT

HOW I'M GOING TO MAKE THIS EASIER FOR MYSELF

MY OWN PLAN

How are you going to change your habits in your day-to-day routine? How are you going to make it easier for yourself in doing so?

NEW HABIT

HOW I'M GOING TO DO IT

HOW I'M GOING TO MAKE THIS EASIER FOR MYSELF

MY OWN PLAN

How are you going to change your habits in your day-to-day routine? How are you going to make it easier for yourself in doing so?

NEW HABIT

HOW I'M GOING TO DO IT

HOW I'M GOING TO MAKE THIS EASIER FOR MYSELF

MY OWN PLAN

How are you going to change your habits in your day-to-day routine? How are you going to make it easier for yourself in doing so?

NEW HABIT

HOW I'M GOING TO DO IT

HOW I'M GOING TO MAKE THIS EASIER FOR MYSELF

MY OWN PLAN

How are you going to change your habits in your day-to-day routine? How are you going to make it easier for yourself in doing so?

NEW HABIT

HOW I'M GOING TO DO IT

HOW I'M GOING TO MAKE THIS EASIER FOR MYSELF

MY OWN PLAN

How are you going to change your habits in your day-to-day routine? How are you going to make it easier for yourself in doing so?

NEW HABIT

HOW I'M GOING TO DO IT

HOW I'M GOING TO MAKE THIS EASIER FOR MYSELF

MY OWN PLAN

How are you going to change your habits in your day-to-day routine? How are you going to make it easier for yourself in doing so?

NEW HABIT

HOW I'M GOING TO DO IT

HOW I'M GOING TO MAKE THIS EASIER FOR MYSELF

MY OWN PLAN

How are you going to change your habits in your day-to-day routine? How are you going to make it easier for yourself in doing so?

NEW HABIT

HOW I'M GOING TO DO IT

HOW I'M GOING TO MAKE THIS EASIER FOR MYSELF

MY OWN PLAN

How are you going to change your habits in your day-to-day routine? How are you going to make it easier for yourself in doing so?

NEW HABIT

HOW I'M GOING TO DO IT

HOW I'M GOING TO MAKE THIS EASIER FOR MYSELF

CHAPTER

04

MONTHLY HABIT TRACKERS

Hold yourself accountable for the next 12 months of your journey. Every day again.

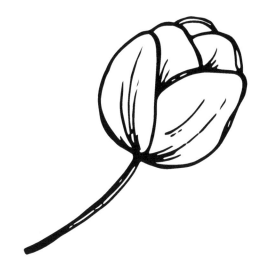

"

BARIATRIC SURGERY ISN'T ABOUT LOSING WEIGHT FAST

IT'S ABOUT CREATING HABITS THAT LAST

-
YOUR ONEDERLAND

INSTRUCTIONS

Using a habit tracker

You now have identified which habits you want to work on. That's great! You're already in the motion of change. In the pages that follow, you'll see 12 habit trackers to fill in. Use 1 habit tracker for each month.

Your habit tracker helps you to hold yourself accountable*.

Using a habit tracker is a whole new habit on its own! Don't worry if you don't act on your new habit perfectly.

For example, if your new habit is "planning my meals ahead" - and you've looked up a new recipe today, you've actively worked on your new habit. This means that you can tick off one of the boxes in your habit tracker. Keep that streak going!

Remember, it's not about how fast you're changing - but it's all about **moving in the right direction**.

If you missed a day - make it a habit to never skip 2 days in a row. Repetition is key!

Tips for using your habit tracker

Here are 5 tips to make habit tracking more inspiring:

- Use different colors for each habit to create a nicer visual.
- Try not to change too many things all at once: progress over perfection!
- Keep reminding yourself of your "why" (yes - the one you wrote down in the beginning of this journal).
- Reward yourself whenever you hit a new milestone. For example, whenever you have a 7-day "habit streak" give yourself a small gift to celebrate.
- Be specific with the habits you write down. For example, "being healthy" is too broad. So why not start with "taking my vitamins every day". And break it down into smaller routines that support your long-term goal.

Are you ready to get started? Let's do this!

*If you want more accountability in the form of a daily planner - you can learn more about our bariatric planner collection here: www.youronederland.com/bariplanner

-79-

AN EXAMPLE

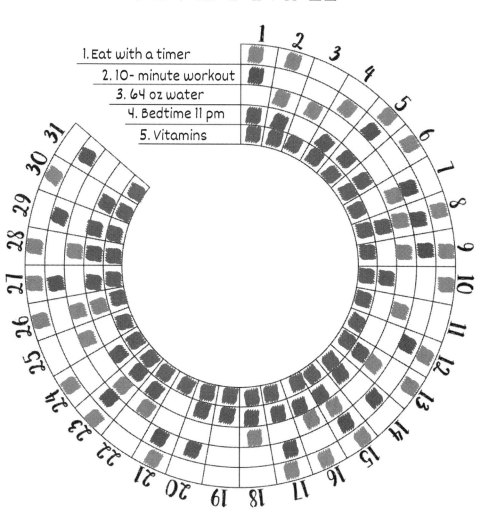

1. Eat with a timer
2. 10- minute workout
3. 64 oz water
4. Bedtime 11 pm
5. Vitamins

MY NOTES

....

....

....

MONTH 1

Month of:
....

1 2 3 4 5 6 7 8 9 10 11 12 13 14 15 16 17 18 19 20 21 22 23 24 25 26 27 28 29 30 31

MY NOTES

....

....

....

MONTH 2

Month of:
....

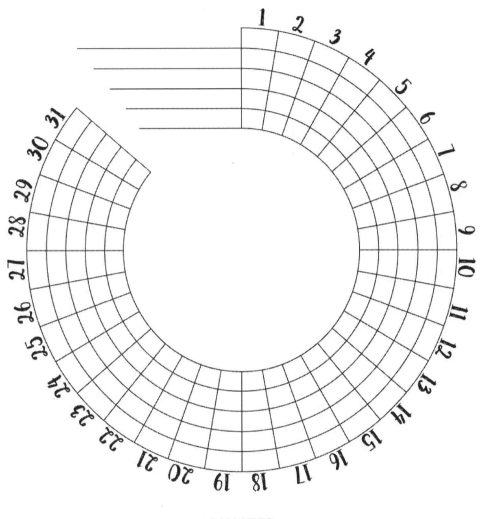

MY NOTES

....

....

....

MONTH 3

Month of: ....

MY NOTES

....

....

....

MONTH 4

Month of: ....

MY NOTES

....

....

....

MONTH 5

Month of:
....

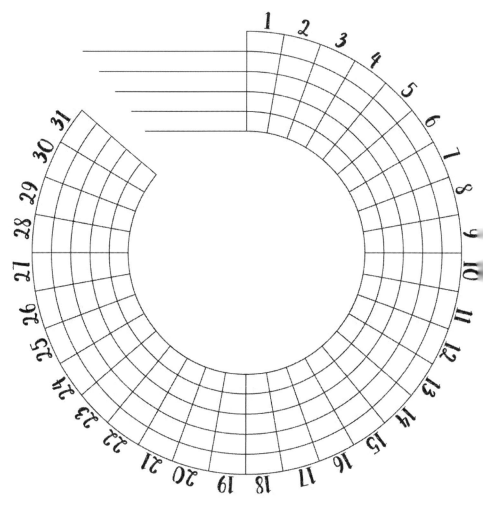

MY NOTES

....

....

....

MONTH 6

Month of: ....

MY NOTES

....

....

....

MONTH 7

Month of: ....

1 2 3 4 5 6 7 8 9 10 11 12 13 14 15 16 17 18 19 20 21 22 23 24 25 26 27 28 29 30 31

MY NOTES

....

....

....

MONTH 8

Month of: ....

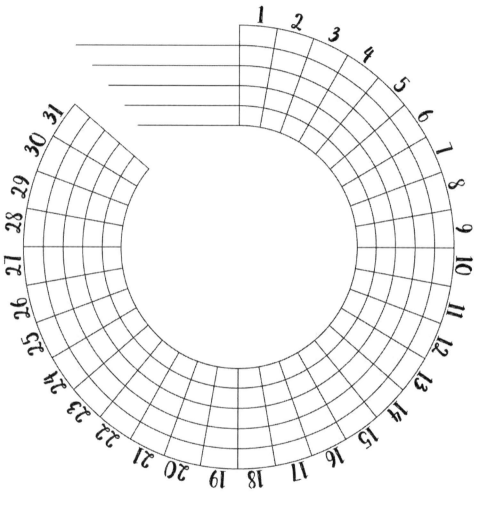

MY NOTES

....

....

....

MONTH 9

Month of:

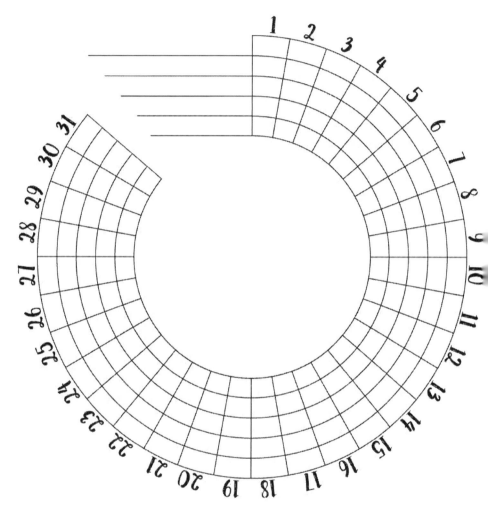

MY NOTES

MONTH 10

Month of: ....

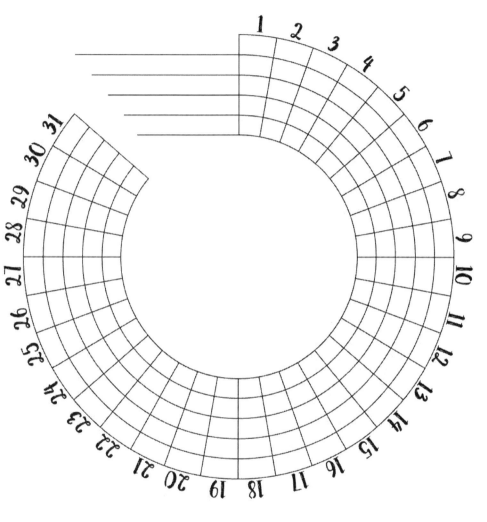

MY NOTES

....

....

....

MONTH 11

Month of: ....

MY NOTES

....

....

....

MONTH 12

Month of:

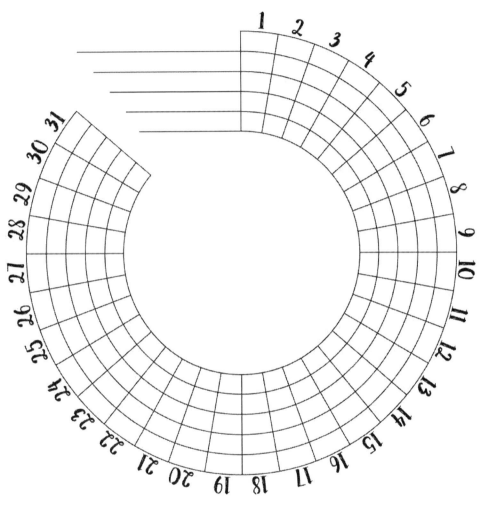

MY NOTES

CHAPTER

05

QUARTERLY PROGRESS CHARTS

Celebrate your wins - on and off the scale - with these progress charts.

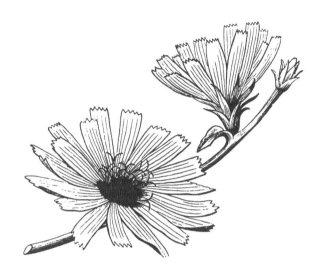

"

BARIATRIC SURGERY ISN'T A COMPETITION

IT'S ABOUT YOU WINNING YOUR OWN RACE

-

YOUR ONEDERLAND

MONTH 3 PROGRESS CHART

Weight Loss Progress

Highest
Weight:

3 months
post-op:

Total
Lost:

My Milestones

- 🎗 _____
- 🎗 _____
- 🎗 _____
- 🎗 _____
- 🎗 _____
- 🎗 _____
- 🎗 _____

Total in/cm Lost

Favorite Meal

_____

Greatest Challenge

_____

Happiest Moment

_____

I'm going to be more mindful in the next 3 months about:

_____

_____

MONTH 6 PROGRESS CHART

Weight Loss Progress

Highest
Weight:

6 months
post-op:

Total
Lost:

My Milestones

_____

_____

_____

_____

_____

_____

_____

Total in/cm Lost

Favorite Meal

_____

Greatest Challenge

_____

Happiest Moment

_____

I'm going to be more mindful in the next 3 months about:

_____

_____

MONTH 9 PROGRESS CHART

Weight Loss Progress

Highest
Weight:

9 months
post-op:

Total
Lost:

My Milestones

Ⓡ _____

Ⓡ _____

Ⓡ _____

Ⓡ _____

Ⓡ _____

Ⓡ _____

Ⓡ _____

Total in/cm Lost

Favorite Meal
_____

Greatest Challenge
_____

Happiest Moment
_____

I'm going to be more mindful in the next **3** months about:

_____

_____

MONTH 12 PROGRESS CHART

Weight Loss Progress

Highest
Weight:

12 months
post-op:

Total
Lost:

My Milestones

- _____
- _____
- _____
- _____
- _____
- _____
- _____

Total in/cm Lost

Favorite Meal

_____

Greatest Challenge

_____

Happiest Moment

_____

I'm going to be more mindful in the next 3 months about:

_____

_____

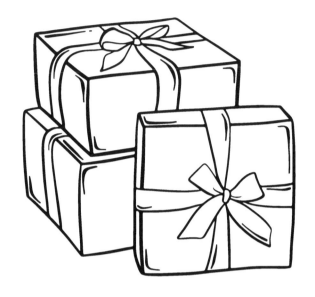

"

YOU'VE MADE IT THIS FAR ALREADY. REMEMBER THAT.

-

YOUR ONEDERLAND

HERE'S WHAT TO DO NEXT

Congratulations on making it to the end of this journal. You now have a new set of habits to continue to work on (remember, there's no finish line in this journey - but a life-long commitment to keep improving yourself). But what's next? What can you do to stay on the right track? No worries, we've got answers!

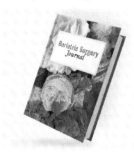 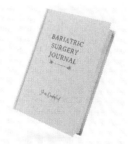 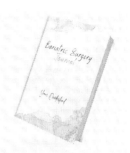

REDEFINE THE NEXT 8 WEEKS OF YOUR JOURNEY

Don't let your new mindset go to waste. You've worked so incredibly hard to keep the promise you made to yourself many months ago. To live your best life possible.

Now imagine that all your hard work would crumble away? What if you lose your focus - and you feel yourself slipping back into old habits again?

Be smart - and use the Bariatric Surgery Journal from Your Onederland to keep yourself accountable for the next 8 weeks of your journey.

This Bariatric Surgery Journal has all the tools you need to make sure you never lose sight of the bariatric basics again.

Learn more about our journals and planners here:

www.youronederland.com/bariplanner

GET THE SUPPORT YOU DESERVE

Did you know that there's a whole community out there filled with bariatric resources to make sure that you have tips that actually work? A community with its own social platform where meaningful connections are made every single day? With thousands of bariatric friends joined worldwide - we're welcoming you to join our squad too!

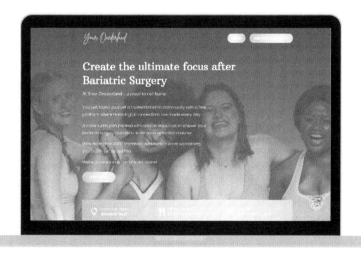

Learn more about our bariatric community here:

www.youronederland.com/about-our-community

WE'RE A COMMUNITY - YOU'RE NOT ALONE!

-xoxo- Your Onederland

Made in the USA
Las Vegas, NV
06 August 2023

75699618R10059